A CONCISE GUIDE TO LOSE YOUR BELLY DIET

Change your life, improve your health, lose your belly and get rid of those sugar cravings forever

Thomas W. Gil

Disclaimer

This book is intended to provide accurate, dependable information about the issue at hand. The author's thoughts in this work, on the other side, are solely his or her own and should not be construed as professional instruction or guidance. The reader is accountable for his or her actions. The author expressly states that he or she is not liable for the way the buyer and reader apply the material in this book. The individual who purchases or reads the material accepts complete responsibility for his or her actions.

Every right is intact. Without the express permission of the publisher, no part of this book may be copied, duplicated, or reproduced in any manner, including copying, recording, or even other mechanical or electronic techniques. Short extracts used during reviews and some nonprofit uses permitted by copyright rules are the sole exceptions. Please contact the publisher just at the address shown below to request authorization.

TABLE OF CONTENTS

INTRODUCTION

By the World Health Organization, approximately 1.9 billion persons were overweight and obese in 2016. Keeping a healthy lifestyle may be tough if your life is hectic and stressful. Many causes, including stress, bad eating, technology reliance, a sedentary lifestyle, and easy access to fast food, have all contributed to belly obesity. Belly fat is among the most difficult fats to lose. To get treatment for stubborn belly fat, you need a long-term, healthy regimen. Making simple adjustments in your life may have a big impact on your total weight and belly fat. A rise in belly fat may suggest a variety of health concerns, including diabetes, heart disease, and liver damage. Men's and women's bodies react differently to abdominal fat. While belly fat in males causes cardiovascular disease, disease resistance, and high blood pressure, Harvard Health Publishing reports that belly fat in women is more dangerous. A hip-to-waist and BMI study reveals that women had an 18% higher likelihood of having a heart attack than males. In women, it may also raise the risk of developing diabetes and breast cancer.

WHAT IS BELLY FAT?

A potentially hazardous form of fat that covers organs in the abdomen is known as abdomen, stomach, or belly fat. For some individuals, reducing belly fat might have considerable health advantages.

Belly fat produces hormones that may cause type-2 diabetes, heart disease, and other health issues. Due to its active function in the production of numerous hormones, it is frequently referred to as "active fat."

This fat is less apparent than fat deposits, which are found immediately under the skin. A visible rise in waist circumference, on the other hand, might indicate an increase in visceral fat.

Visceral fat is very sensitive to how a person consumes. Making important dietary modifications and engaging in the appropriate types of exercise may help to decrease this sort of fat.

FACTORS CONTRIBUTE TO BELLY FAT

Diet, inadequate exercise, environmental circumstances, and heredity are all variables that contribute to abdominal fat.

Surplus Calories

The most prevalent cause of abdominal obesity is poor diet. While it's tempting to blame one single food type or ingredient, such as sugar or carbohydrates, for excess weight, the truth is that the total calories consumed each day are the true cause. Finding the balance between exercising your body and appropriately fueling it (for the amount of exercise you're doing) may be challenging no matter what you eat. Furthermore, a sedentary lifestyle needs fewer calories. As a result, your body does not need to work as difficult to keep yourself going. Because the human body prefers to conserve energy, this will slow down when no energy is required, such as when you devote more time resting than doing anything else.

Metabolism

It's simple to blame weight gain on a slow metabolism. While this may be accurate for some, it is not true for others. If fat reduction is your objective, there are easy techniques to boost your metabolism. Metabolism encompasses all of the processes through which the body turns fuel into energy. These procedures are as follows:

Metabolic processes include:

- Breathing
- Blood circulation
- Body temperature regulation
- Muscle contraction
- Food and nutrient digestion
- Waste removal by pee and feces
- The operation of the brain

Your metabolism might be rapid, slow, or moderate; this is mostly determined by heredity. When you have a sluggish metabolism, it might be disheartening to attempt to lose weight and find that it isn't falling off as readily as it used to. Then some individuals seem to have a rapid metabolism and can eat anything they want without gaining a pound.

Age has an impact on metabolism as well. As we become older, our metabolism slows down. Many individuals become less active, resulting in a loss of lean body mass (muscle). Muscle is a metabolically active tissue that needs energy to sustain itself. Because you have lesser muscles and move less, your metabolism may slow down to compensate.

The fact is that metabolism accounts for just a minor portion of what drives weight gain. Understanding your metabolism and how to enhance it can help you avoid gaining stomach fat over time.

Genetics and Body Fat Distribution

Unfortunately, you have no control over where your body accumulates fat. Some individuals are predisposed to retain fat in their midsections, whereas others store it throughout their bodies. In the same way, you can't choose where you lose weight.

If you're aware of what to anticipate as you get older, you may assist lessen your chances of gaining belly fat.

indicated that menopause is related to weight gain and an increase in abdominal fat distribution Changes in body weight are also caused by chronological aging, however, changes in the body's structure and abdominal obesity are caused by ovarian aging, according to the researchers.

Environmental influences influence how our genes react. Because we don't know when our next meal will be, our bodies are prone to retain fat. That biological desire may now be acting against us, according to the "thrifty genotype" idea.

People often restrict their food consumption to lose weight. If you follow a reduced diet for an extended time, your body will experience food shortage but will slow down or accumulate extra fat. This is the polar opposite of what people who restrict their calorie intake generally want.

Then there's "familial predisposition," which means that the weight of a child's family members might predict their chances of becoming fat.

Hormones

Abdominal fat growth is also linked to fluctuations and changes in a person's hormonal health.

Low-growth hormonal changes caused by hyperinsulinemia and elevated cardiovascular risk indicators may enhance visceral fat formation due to decreased lipolysis sensitivity in this location.

It is also thought that when body fat or leptin levels rise, the quantity of leptin absorbed across the blood-brain membrane decreases, lowering the signals that regulate body weight. However, even though leptin or obesity have been researched for over 25 years, it is still unclear how they are associated.

Mental Wellness

Physical and psychological strain may also contribute to abdominal fat. When you are stressed, your body secretes cortisol, the stress hormone that induces fat storage. increased cortisol levels move adipose tissue to the stomach area and enhance hunger with a predilection for high energy-dense meals, such as comfort foods.

Other studies have shown that high cortisol levels over time are "highly associated" with abdominal fat.

This association also works the other way, as increasing belly fat generally results in higher cortisol, starting a weight-cycling cycle.

Weight increase is also connected to several mental health issues. Obesity is 60% in patients with bipolar illness and schizophrenia, according to studies. 13 Weight gain may be caused by both the mental disorder and the medications taken to treat it.

Medication

Weight gain is a typical adverse effect of many drugs. Diabetes drugs, such as insulin and sulfonylureas, as well as antihypertensive medicines, beta-blockers, corticosteroids, or medications for mood disorders, melancholy, and other mental conditions, have all been linked to weight gain.

TYPES OF BELLY FAT

In comparison to the rest of the body, the belly has very little fat. There are two forms of belly fat: one beneath your skin and one deeper within your abdomen, encompassing your internal organs.

Subcutaneous belly fat

Subcutaneous fat, also known as subcutaneous adipose tissues (SAT), is fat located under the skin.

Fat tissue is soft and is the fact that seems to "jiggle" on your abdomen. Women, on average, have more subcutaneous fat than males.

Subcutaneous fat, as opposed to fat located deeper in the abdominal wall, is not as closely connected to increased disease risk.

Having too much body fat in general, management excellence belly fat may raise your chance of acquiring chronic illnesses such as diabetes type 2 heart disease, and some malignancies.

Maintaining appropriate amounts of belly fat or general body fat, on the other hand, may help minimize your chance of acquiring a chronic condition.

Visceral belly fat

Visceral adipose tissue (VAT), often known as visceral belly fat, is fat that surrounds inner organs such as the kidney, liver, and pancreas, and is located far deeper in your abdomen than subcutaneous fat. This is frequently known as "harmful" abdominal fat.

Visceral fat is substantially more metabolically active than subcutaneous fat. Subcutaneous fat includes fewer cells, arteries, and nerves than this form of fat.

Visceral fat is significantly connected to increased insulin resistance, which controls blood sugar levels. Insulin deficiency may lead to high levels of blood sugar and the formation of diabetes type 2 over time.

Visceral fat also adds to the inflammatory process, which increases the risk of illness.

Men are more prone than women to store visceral fat, resulting in men being more likely to have an "apple-shaped" body when belly fat accumulates. Women, in contrast, hand, are more prone to gain extra fat in their lower bodies, resulting in a "pear" appearance.

Surprisingly, the distribution of body fat alters with age. Premenopausal women, for example, have larger amounts of cutaneous belly fat, but postmenopausal women have greater concentrations of visceral fat, which correlates to an elevated risk of metabolic illness.

Furthermore, visceral fat is greater in persons of European heritage than in those of other races.

MEASUREMENT OF BELLY FAT

Because abdominal obesity puts you at a higher risk for a variety of medical issues, measuring waist circumference may help you understand where you stand.

How to Take Waist Circumference Measurements?

Place the tape measure around the midsection, slightly above your hip bones, while standing.

- Make certain that the tape is straight around your waist.
- Maintain a tight fit around the waist without squeezing the skin.
- Take your waist measurement just after you exhale.

If your waist measurement is greater than the suggested values shown below, it might be time to consult with a medical expert about any potential health problems.

Limits on waist circumference:

- **Male:** more than 40 inches
- **Female:** more than 35 inches

The waist-to-hip proportion is another technique to assess your risk of heart disease as well as other chronic conditions. Recently, the midriff ratio has been criticized since, whereas waist circumference is linked to an increased risk of heart disease, hip size is not.

DANGEROUS ABDOMINAL FAT

Visceral fat has been linked to metabolic illnesses such as meets, type 2 diabetes, heart disease, and specific malignancies such as prostate, belly, and colorectal cancer. Carrying extra fat around your waist, in particular, raises your risk of significant health problems.

Visceral Fat's Potential Dangers

- Mortality from any cause
- Cardiovascular illness

- Cancers of certain kinds

- Their blood pressure is high.

- LDL ("bad") cholesterol levels are elevated.

- Low levels of HDL ("good") cholesterol

- Obstructive sleep apnea

- Diabetes type 2

This is naturally frightening. Take a long, deep breath. Just because you are heavy in the abdomen does not guarantee you will have a chronic health issue.

HOW TO GET RID OF BELLY FAT

There is no one-size-fits-all technique for losing weight. You also can't spot a decrease. However, you may use a variety of tactics to decrease belly fat. Before starting any new weight-reduction plan, always with your doctor.

Consume a Nutritious and Balanced Diet

It is not as easy as decreasing calories to lose belly fat. While a caloric deficit is often required to lose weight, finding out how to do so while discovering what works for you is critical. Working with a licensed dietitian helps you learn what works best for your body and build a balanced, nutritious eating routine that will help you achieve your objectives. no matter what sort of diet you pick, you may have the same fat-reduction outcomes. Within this sense, the greatest diet is one that doesn't seem like a nutrition food pattern that you can keep to is critical for weight control sustainability.

To feel extra full and satisfied, eat complex carbohydrates (including whole grain, fruits, and veggies), protein (like chicken, cattle, milk, egg, fish, and soy), and good fats (like avocados, canola oil, nuts, olives, and nut jars of butter) for breakfast, lunch, and supper. Don't be scared to incorporate a few of your favorite meals to avoid feeling deprived.

Finally, striking a good balance that does not exclude whole food categories or foods is best for sustainable weight reduction.

Include Exercise in Your Daily Routine

Exercise may help you maintain a healthy weight. The CDC advises that persons aged 18 to 64 engage in at least 150 minutes of moderate-intensity physical activity per week, such as walking, as well as at least one or two sessions each week of strength training.

Finding a workout that you love is essential. However, studies suggest that doing an aerobic activity at a moderate to low intensity at least 2 times a week burns less visceral fat than just changing your dietary patterns. looked at the benefits of low-intensity aerobic exercise and strength training on visceral fat reduction and found that both groups saw improvements, but the strength training group had faster results.

Aim to combine both weight-bearing strength training sessions and cardio exercises into your weekly regimen to make the most of the time and training efforts.

Find Stress-Relieving Activities

Stress management is essential not only for your mental health but also for your physical health. We already understand that stress and visceral obesity are linked. Finding techniques to reduce stress daily will assist improve many parts of your life, including your risk of illness. Mindfulness, meditation, breathing methods, yoga, sports, and any other activity that makes you feel good are all stress management strategies. This might be as easy as listening to their favorite music for 10 minutes every day, cuddling up on the sofa with a nice book, or relaxing in a Jacuzzi at night.

Get Plenty of Sleep

Sleep deprivation may be harmful to weight reduction. Around 35percent of Americans report receiving less than eight hours of sleep each night, and 50% report feeling drowsy at least 3 days per week. Adults should sleep for at least 7 hours every night, according to the Centers for Disease Prevention and Prevention. A 2014 research discovered that a lack of sleep might encourage individuals to pick high-calorie and high-carbohydrate diets, which can lead to weight gain.

Furthermore, a lack of sleep may cause key brain chemicals involved in appetite promotion and satiety control to go out of balance.

Set up your sleeping environment for success by doing the following:

How to Create the Perfect Sleep Environment?

- The optimal sleeping temperature is 65 degrees Fahrenheit.

- Loud sounds may interfere with sleep; use a white noise generator and ambient sound to drown out outside noise.
- Maintain the lowest feasible light levels.
- Avoid using displays in your bedroom, especially TVs.
- Choose pillows, mattresses, and bedding that will keep you cool and comfy.
- A clean atmosphere promotes greater sleep.
- Lavender, peppermint, or heliotrope are all relaxing smells to try.

Seek Assistance

A support network is essential for success when beginning any endeavor, including weight reduction. Support may take many forms hiring a trustworthy healthcare expert to help you through this process is a good place to start.

If you feel comfortable doing so, telling your family and friends about your objectives might assist with accountability and encouragement. Finding social groups, whether online or in person, is an excellent method of feeling connected and encouraged.

Doing out with a companion is a terrific way to keep inspired and may even encourage you to exercise extra if you're just starting.

BELLY FAT FOR WOMEN

Visceral fat, and belly fat, that accumulates around internal organs may raise a woman's risk of developing diabetes or heart disease. Fortunately, visceral fat is biologically active and may be swiftly decreased with a focused mix of diet, exercise, and stress reduction. You may reduce belly fat quickly by controlling stress hormones & increasing your metabolism.

Eating with Intention

1. As the saying goes, "abs are created in the kitchen."

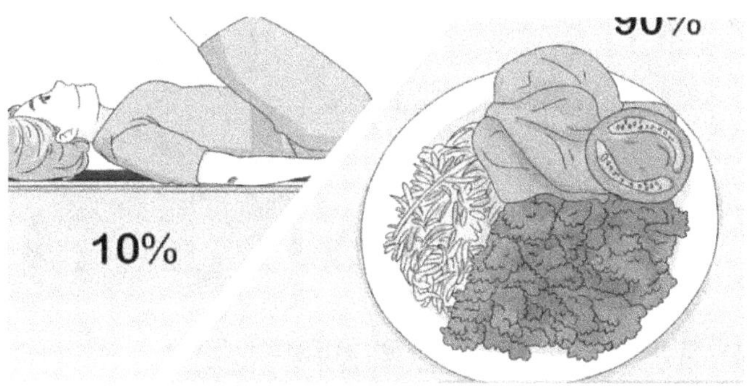

According to most personal trainers, decreasing belly fat involves 90% nutrition and 10% exercise. This step is critical if you do not consume a well-balanced diet.

2. Eliminate processed sugars and carbohydrates.

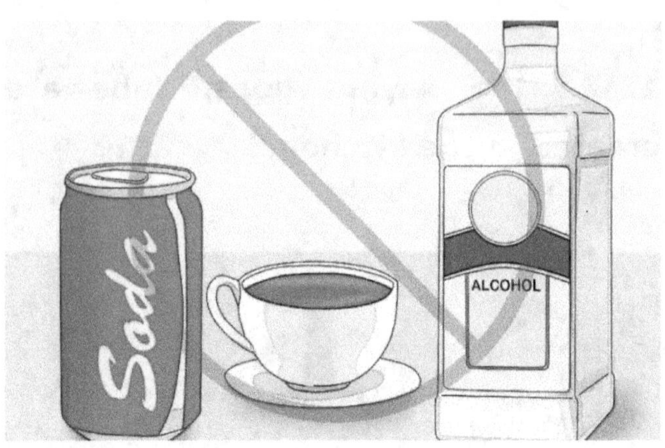

Reducing the amount of sugar + empty calories in white processed carbs can help you burn fat quicker. This includes liquid calories such as soda, coffee, and alcohol. Most dietitians believe that eliminating processed meals is the only way to decrease belly fat swiftly and healthfully.

3. Plan your meals around fruit and vegetable portions.

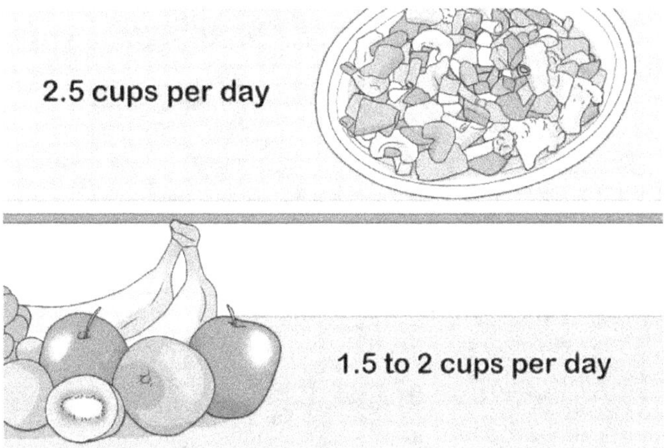

A woman aged 19 to 50 needs at least 2.5 cups of veggies each day. Color is important when selecting veggies. Making a bright dish can help you receive more nutrients. Women aged 19 to 50 should consume 1.5 to 2 cups of fruit every day. *Eating your favorite fruits can help increase your appetite for nutritious meals.

4. Include entire grains.

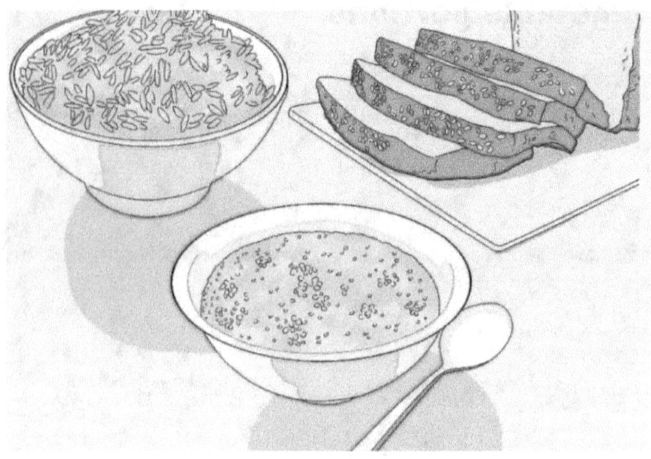

 Over whole-grain bread, choose grains like quinoa, brown rice, and barley. The less processed the grain, the healthier your body will be.

Select whole grains with a low glycemic index. This means they won't cause a rise in your blood sugar and will keep you fuller for longer.

To see how your favorite foods, rank on the glycemic index, go to glycemicindex.com.

5. Prepare your protein.

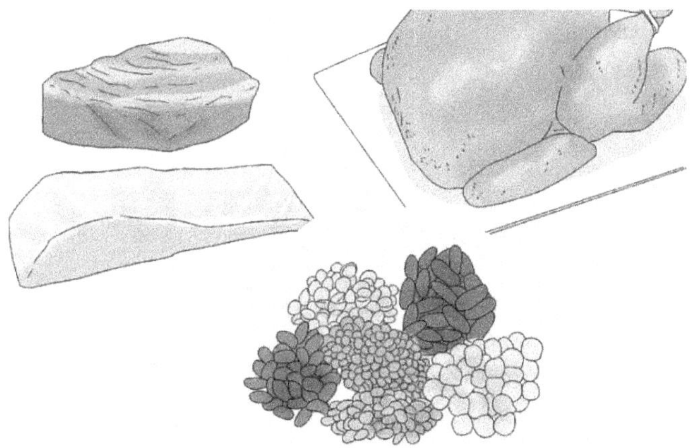

Every day, consume high-quality protein such as salmon, tuna, turkey, chicken, and lentils (women who are pregnant, nursing, or considering getting pregnant should be careful about the amount of mercury in their diet and avoid eating excessive quantities of some fish). Yogurt is a good source of low-fat dairy. Yogurt contains calcium, which helps reduce cortisol levels. Greek yogurt has more protein than normal yogurt, and eating one serving per day as part of a balanced diet will help you lose belly fat quicker.

6. Drink 2–5 cups of green tea every day.

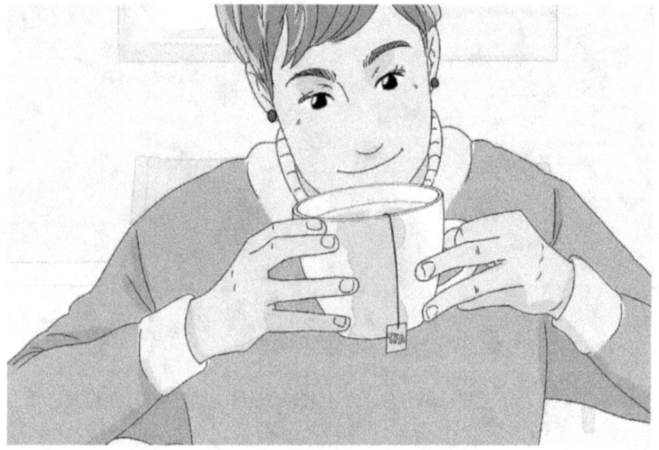

According to studies, participants who consumed 600mg of catechins, an antioxidant contained in green tea, shed 16 times more visceral fat than those who did not.

Look for green tea with strong anti-oxidant content.

To get these advantages, you must consume it hot.

Strategic Exercising

1. Do 1 hour of cardio activity every day to lose weight quickly.

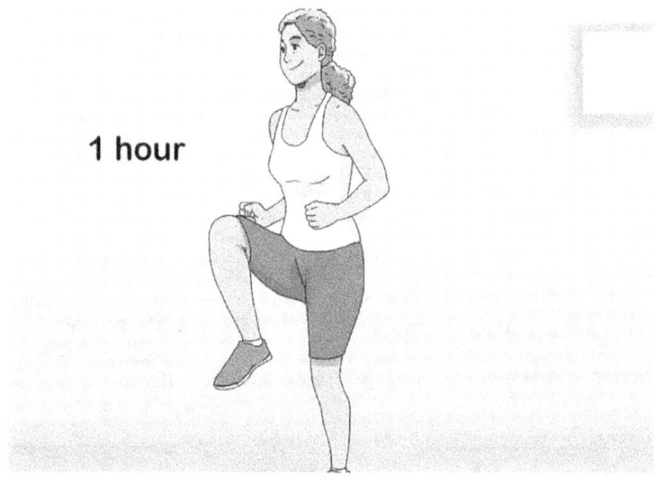

Although 30 minutes of moderate cardiac activity per day may block the development of new visceral fat, it takes an hour to burn it. You cannot "spot reduce," or burn stomach fat just, without also reducing other body fat. However, 90% of individuals initially perceive a decrease in abdominal fat.

2. Choose interval training.

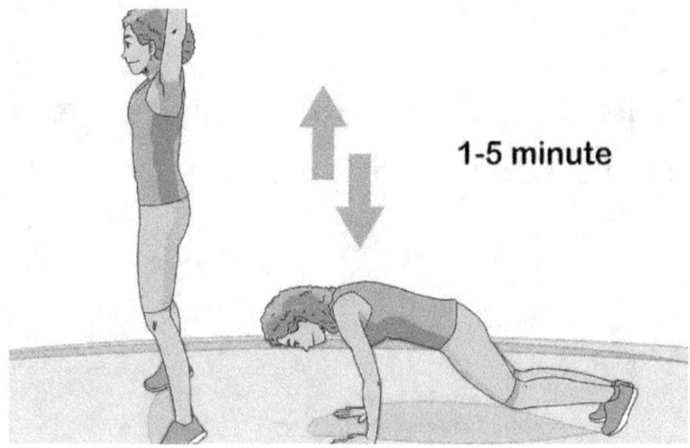

Short bursts of high-intensity exercise (1-5 minutes) within a 1-hour session can enhance your metabolism and help you lose weight faster.

To learn how to include high-intensity activities into your regimen, enroll in a boot camp, circuit training, or fat-burning class.

Interval settings may also be found on most cardiovascular devices.

3. Perform bodyweight workouts before conventional crunches.

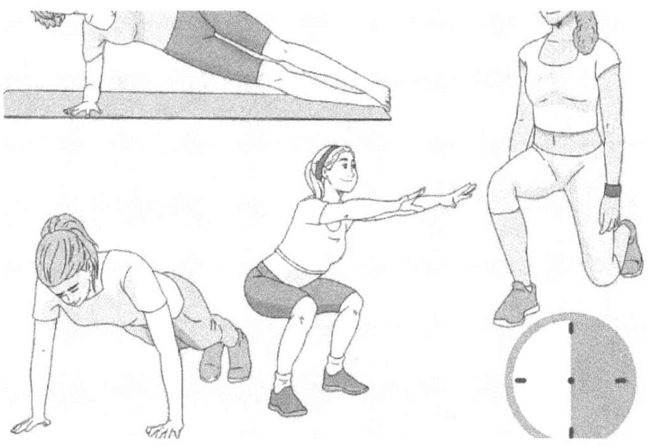

Every other day, do planks, side planks, push-ups, squats, and lunges.

Every other day, try to integrate 30 minutes of bodyweight workouts.

Because they activate your core muscles, such as the abdominals, for a longer and more intense time, these static and dynamic exercises burn more fat than crunches.

When your body has adapted to the increased activity, including strength training using machines or free weights. 3 times a week, perform 30 minutes of weightlifting with your abs flexed.

4. Stretch your abs before working out.

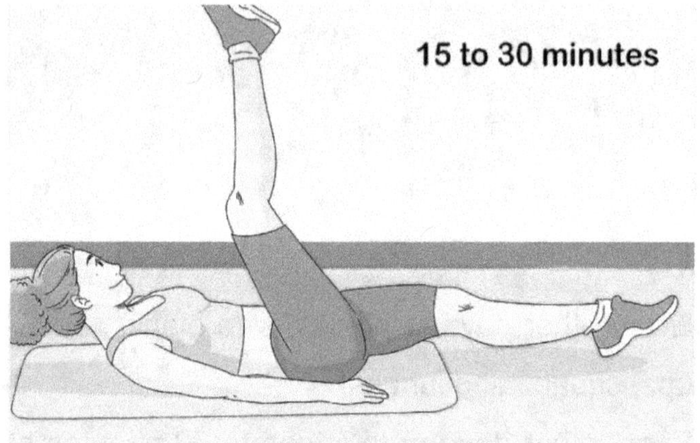

Try to perform your cardio before you do your abdominal workouts and stretches so that your core gets more attention than your tight hips, legs, or neck.

Learn how to target the deep abdominal muscles by taking a Pilates session.

Every other day, perform 15 to 30 minutes of abdominal exercises.

Include workouts that target the obliques (side abs) and transverse abdominis (lower abs). Side plank dips, reverse crunches, the bicycle, and roll-downs are all good workouts.

If you had a C-section, see your doctor before engaging in any activity.

Stress Hormone Balance

1. Determine the sources of stress in your life.

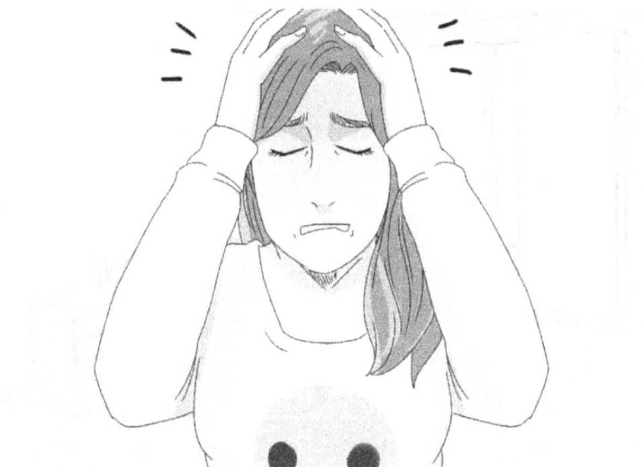

In both men and women, stress has been associated with an increase in visceral fat.

When you are stressed, your body produces extra stress chemicals such as cortisol.

Cortisol instructs your body to retain fat. The tension is your body's warning that food may become scarce in the future.

According to several studies, women exhibit higher physical stress indicators than males, including belly fat growth.

2. Reduce stressful circumstances at home and work as soon as possible.

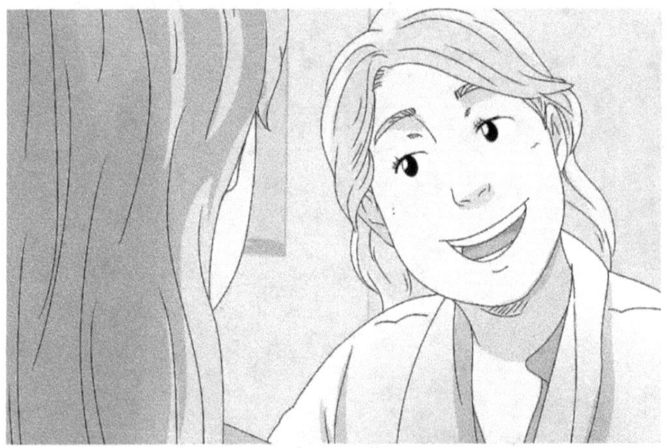

Stress management can help you lose belly fat quicker than diet and exercise alone.

3. Begin practicing deep breathing techniques.

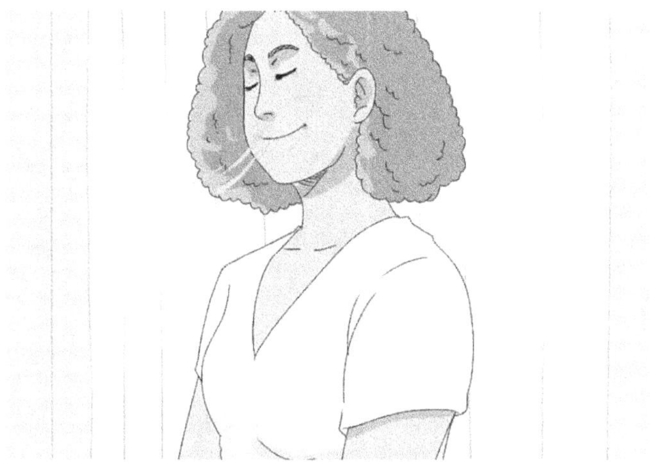

Take ten-second breaths. Place yourself in a comfortable posture. Inhale for 10 seconds, and then exhale for 10 seconds. Breathe in this way for 2 to 5 minutes.

When people are agitated, they tend to breathe quickly in and out and take short breaths without even realizing it.

Breathe for 10 seconds every time you feel agitated, or at 5 different intervals throughout the day.

4. Consider taking vitamin C pills.

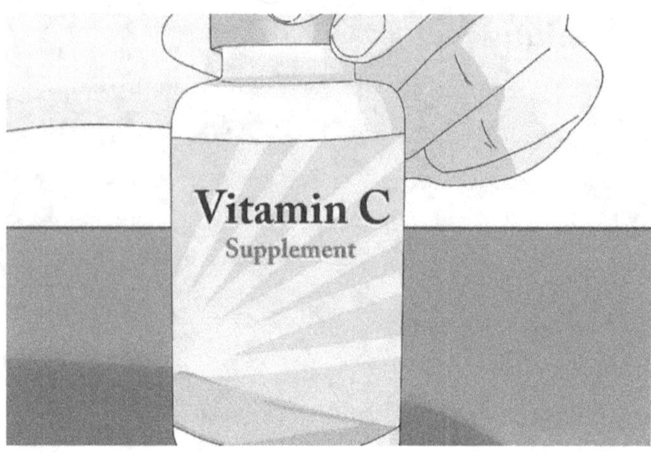

If you don't receive enough Vitamin C through diet, taking a Vitamin C supplement may help you control your cortisol levels and the effects of stress on your body.

Try to consume more melon, oranges, red and green peppers, kiwi, broccoli, or tomatoes. A serving of each offer between 40 and 100mg of Vitamin C.

Consume 500mg of vitamin C every day. Make an effort to receive the bulk of your Vitamin C through food.

If you aren't getting your 500mg of Vitamin C, take a 200mg supplement. If you believe you are not receiving enough Vitamin C in your diet, you may take a 500mg supplement for a week.

5. Sleep for 7 to 8 hours every night.

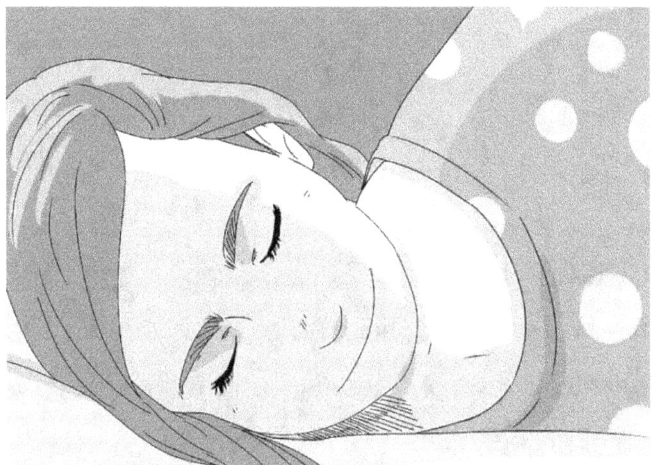

Sleeping properly helps to control stress and hormone levels.

Sleeping fewer than 7 hours every day might increase cortisol and ghrelin levels, leading you to accumulate belly fat.

Ghrelin is a hormone that causes sweet and fatty food cravings.

6. Attempt yoga or meditation.

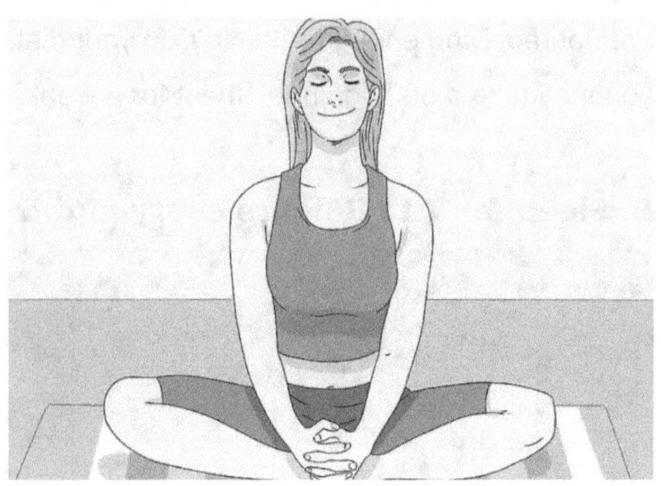

If deep breathing is assisting, yoga and meditation could be the greatest strategy to balance cortisol, ghrelin, and other weight-gaining chemicals.

To reduce belly fat quickly, try several styles of yoga for fitness and stress reduction. Flowing yoga burns fat and relieves stress.

Meditation may also help you sleep if you attempt it. In addition to greater activity, it should be included in your timetable.

BELLY FAT FOR MEN

Belly fat may be ugly and hard to get rid of, but it is a problem of more than simply looks. Carrying too much weight in your midriff is dangerous, particularly for males. A bigger waist circumference (or measurement around your waistline) increases your risk of many chronic conditions, including diabetes, heart disease, sleep apnea, and even some malignancies (like colon or rectal cancer). Losing weight may help you minimize the amount of abdominal fat you have and the problems it presents. Make a few dietary and lifestyle modifications to help you lose weight and live a healthier life.

Diet Changes to Lose Belly Fat

1. Consult your doctor.

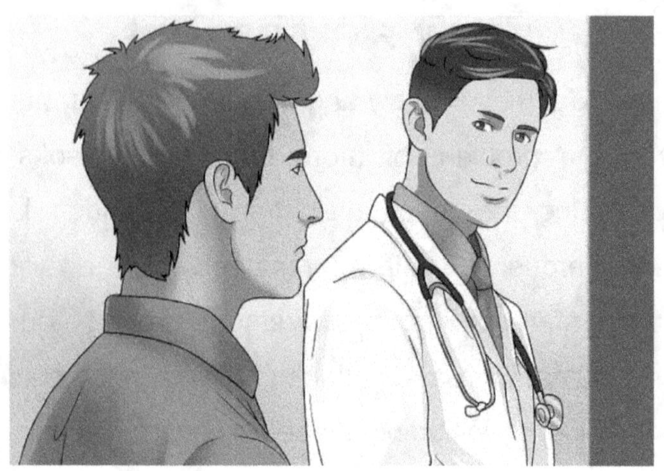

Before beginning any new diet or physical activity program, consult with your doctor. They will be able to inform you if your strategy is safe and suitable for you.

Excess abdominal fat is often linked to a variety of chronic health issues such as diabetes or heart disease. This emphasizes the need of informing your doctor about your strategy and ensuring that it is safe for your health problems.

2. Reduce your carbohydrate intake.

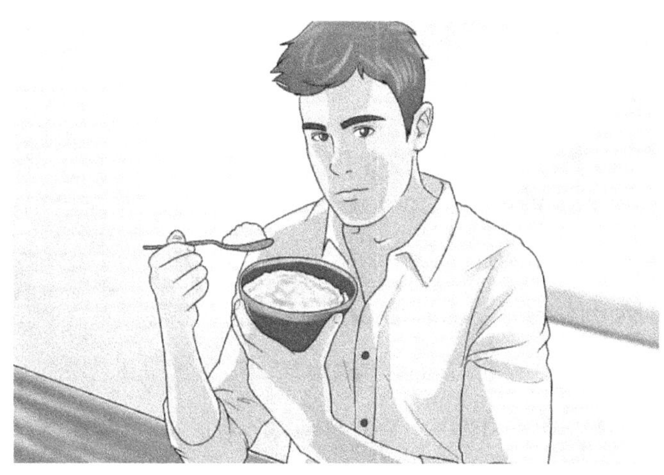

Carbohydrate-rich diets have been demonstrated in studies to increase belly fat and waist circumference. Reduce your intake of these foods to aid in weight loss and the reduction of belly fat. Your diet should mostly consist of lean proteins, vegetables, fruits, and low-fat dairy products.

Limit your consumption of empty carbs such as bread, rice, crackers, and pasta. These foods are not inherently bad, particularly if they are whole grain foods, but they are not nutrient-dense.

If you must have carbohydrates, consider 100% whole grains. These foods are richer in fiber and several minerals, making them a healthier option. Make sure to pay attention to portion sizes as well. One amount of pasta or rice should be half a cup or 125 ml.

Brown rice, 100% whole wheat bread and pasta, barley, and quinoa are examples of whole grain meals.

3. Consume plenty of lean protein.

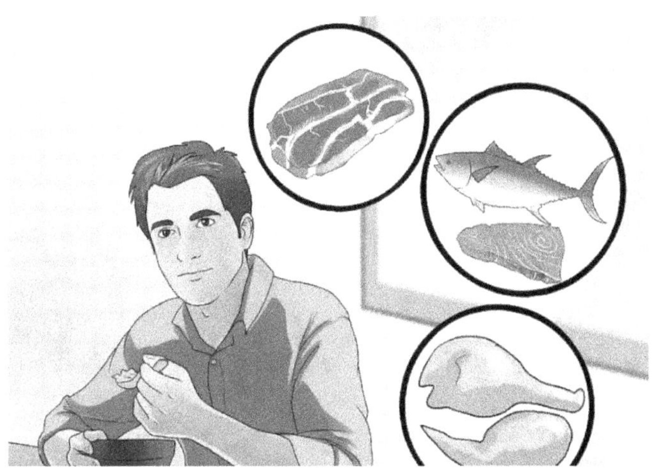

Protein-rich diets may assist men in losing weight, reducing belly fat, and maintaining lean muscle mass. Consuming enough protein can also help you feel full for a longer time.

Protein should account for 20 to 25% of your daily calories if you want to reduce fat. If you eat 1,600 calories each day, you require 80 to 100 grams of protein, if you eat 1,200 calories each day, you need 60 to 75 protein grams.

Lean proteins include lentils, skinless chicken, turkey, egg, low-fat dairy, seafood, pork, lean beef, and tofu. These give you the energy you need while still maintaining your fullness without adding unnecessary calories to your diet.

4. Establish a calorie deficit.

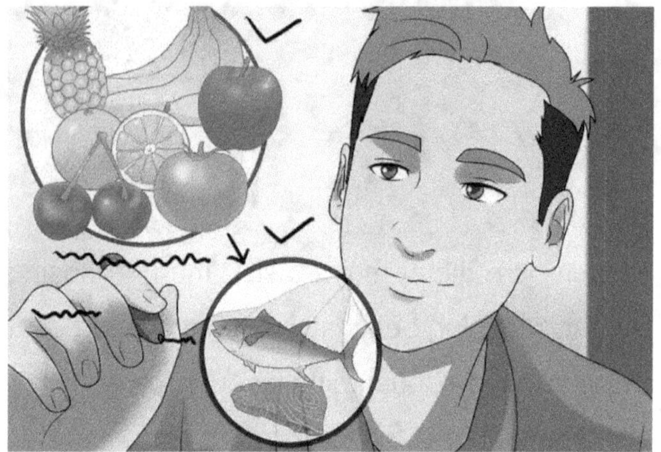

Reduce your overall daily calorie intake to aid in weight loss. You may do this in a variety of ways. Reduce your portion sizes, increase your physical activity, and change the composition of your food to be higher in protein, lower in fat, and lower in carbs.

Begin tracking the number of calories you eat daily. Remember to account for the calories in drinks, cooking oils, salad dressings, and sauces.

Start a food diary to keep track of what you eat. Online food diaries and smartphone applications are intended to assist users in determining the calorie count of the items they consume, keeping track of their consumption, and even connecting with other dieters.

The number of calories you need to consume to lose weight is determined by your age, build, and degree of physical activity. Cut 500 to 1,000 calories each day to lose 1 to 2 pounds per week. This pace of weight reduction is safe and suitable for the majority of guys.

5. Sugar consumption should be reduced.

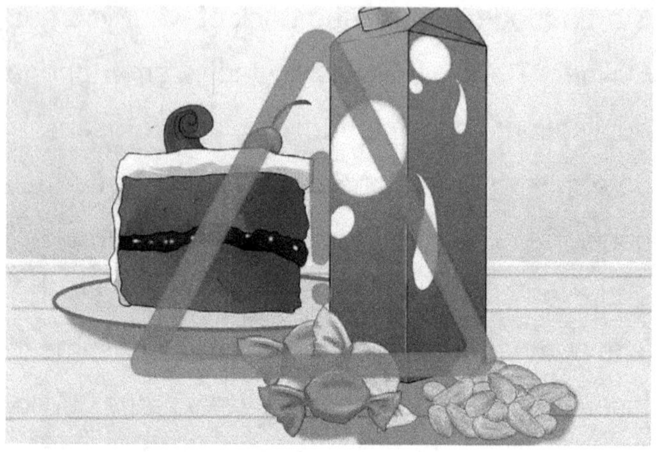

Sugar intake has been linked to an increase in belly fat over time, according to research. Men with a lower sugar intake have a smaller waist circumference.

Sweetened drinks, candies, cookies, cakes, and other sweets, and meals produced with white flour are all items to restrict or avoid (like white bread or plain pasta).

If you're wanting sugar, consider eating a piece of fruit or a little portion of your favorite sweet.

6. Get rid of the booze.

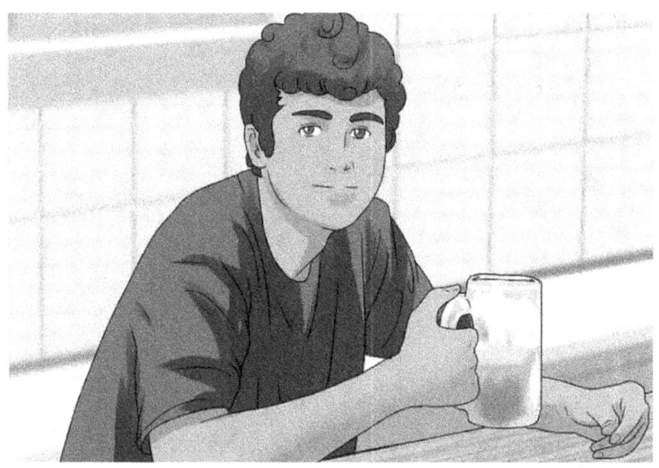

There's a reason it's called a "beer belly," but beer isn't the only beverage that promotes extra belly fat. According to studies, all forms of alcohol might cause belly fat in men.

For males, it is advised that they consume no more than two alcoholic drinks every day; however, if they want to lose belly fat, they should stop drinking entirely.

Physical Activity Can Help You Lose Belly Fat

1. Begin working out.

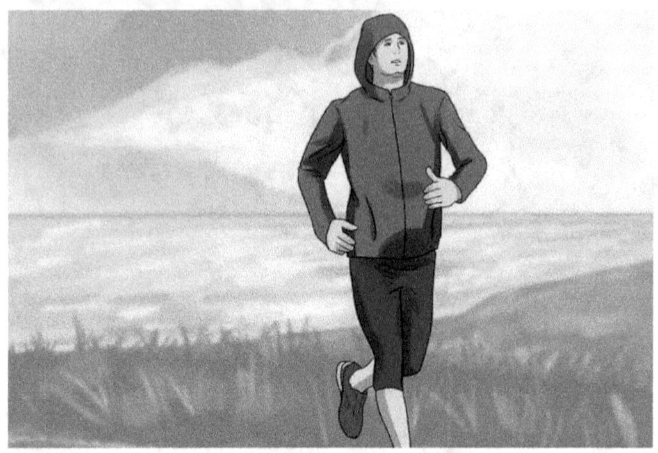

Exercise paired with a low-calorie diet will aid and accelerate weight reduction by burning calories and improving metabolism. Regular cardiovascular exercise might help you lose weight and reduce abdominal fat.

Running, hiking, riding, and swimming are all examples of aerobic workouts that burn calories. For a small benefit, aim for at least 30 minutes of cardiovascular activity five times each week.

Find methods to include more movement into your routine if you don't want to work out every day. Make it a habit to use the stairs instead of the elevator, to park farther away from your destination, and to use a standing workstation. Exercise is particularly vital if you have a sedentary desk job.

2. Regular strength exercises should be included.

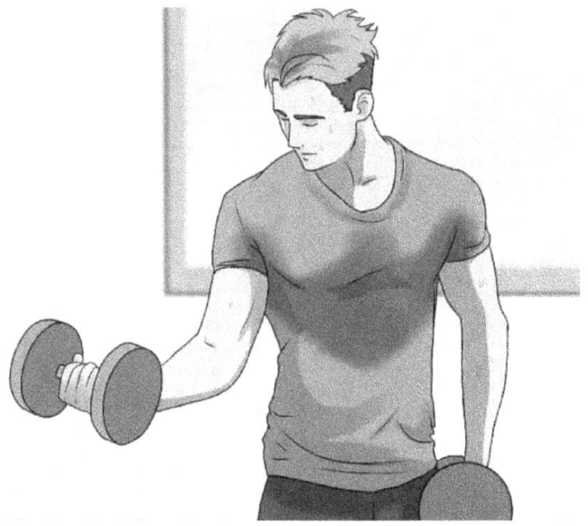

It may get more difficult to lose abdominal fat as you get older. This is due in part to the normal decline in muscle mass as people age, but it is also related to the accumulation of fat around your stomach. Keeping lean muscle mass may assist to avoid this.

Include two days per week of 20 to 30 minutes of weight or resistance exercise.

Weight lifting, weight classes, weight machines, and yoga are all examples of strength training activities.

3. Include workouts for the whole body.

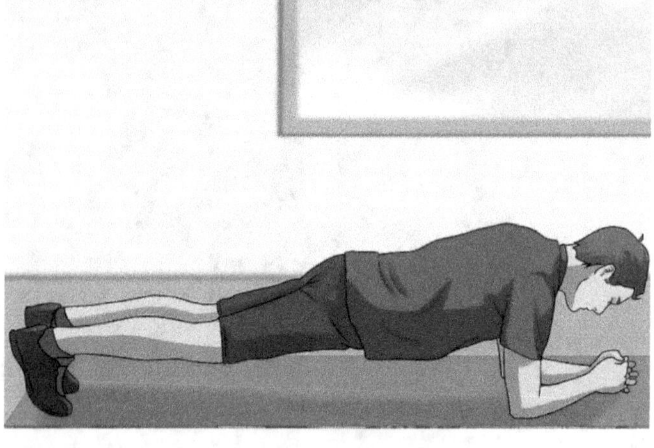

"Spot-training," or concentrating just on movements like crunches and planks, may help strengthen the core, but it will not help you lose belly fat. Toning or strength training activities increase lean muscle mass but do not reduce belly fat.

Concentrate on total weight reduction. Make dietary changes and include adequate quantities of exercise. Then, to tone your abdomen, start including abdominal exercises in your program.

4. Find a workout partner.

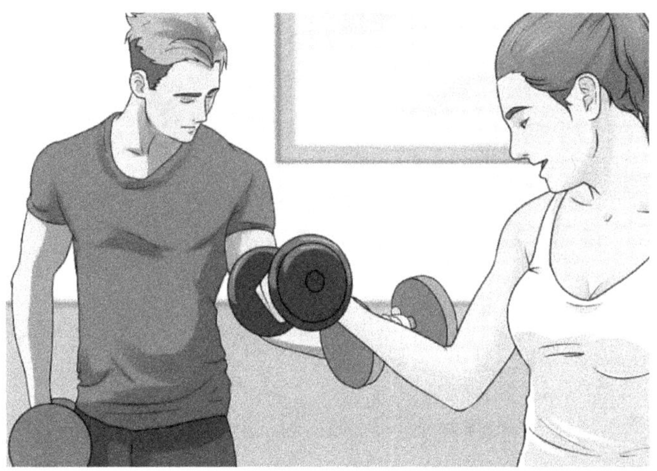

Having someone join you in your exercises might make it more fun. According to research, if you go to the gym with a buddy, you are more likely to stick to your training routine and exercise more often.

If you like competition, you may race your weight-loss friend to see who can achieve their target weight first.

Maintaining Motivation and Tracking Progress

1. Check your weight.

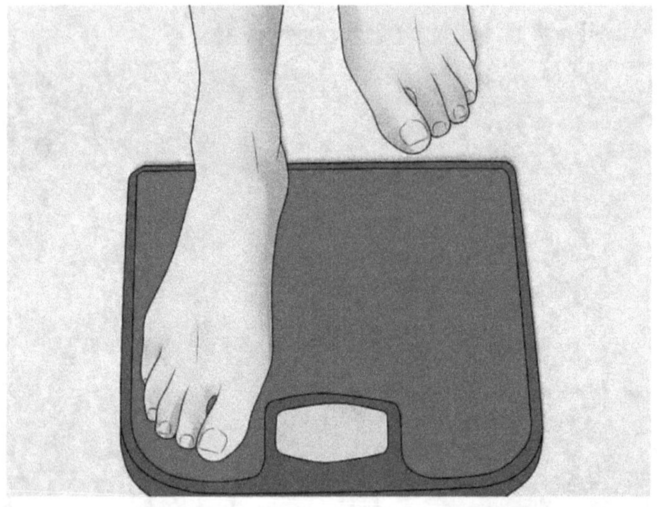

To get rid of or minimize belly fat, you must first lose weight. Weigh yourself regularly to help you keep a record of your weight reduction.

It's advisable to weigh oneself once or twice a week. Furthermore, try to weigh oneself on the same day of the week, at the same hour, and in the same clothing every time.

Keep a notebook to record your weight. Seeing your success might motivate you to remain on track. It may also show them any tendencies in which you are gaining weight.

2. Take some measurements.

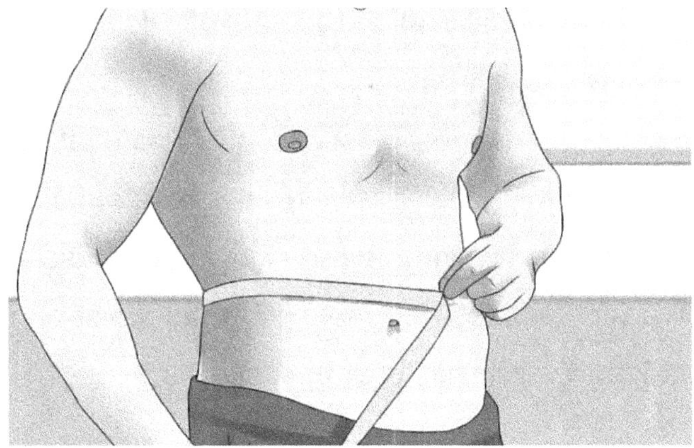

Tracking your waist circumference, in addition to weight reduction, is one of the greatest methods to monitor your progress in decreasing belly fat. This is the circumference of your waist at its narrowest point. Your waist measurement will shrink as you lose abdominal fat.

Measure the length of your waist using a tape measure. Locate the bottom of the hip bone or your lowest rib, then wrap the tape across the belly between such two places. Continue to take measurements while you diet to monitor your improvement.

A big waist circumference, or a measurement of more than 37 inches (94 cm), shows that you have a lot of belly fat and you are at risk for long-term illnesses.

Remember that lean tissue is much more fat, so the scale might be deceiving if you're attempting to reduce weight while growing muscle. Tracking success by measuring the waist and weight combined is your best bet.

3. Prepare a list of alternative activities to eat.

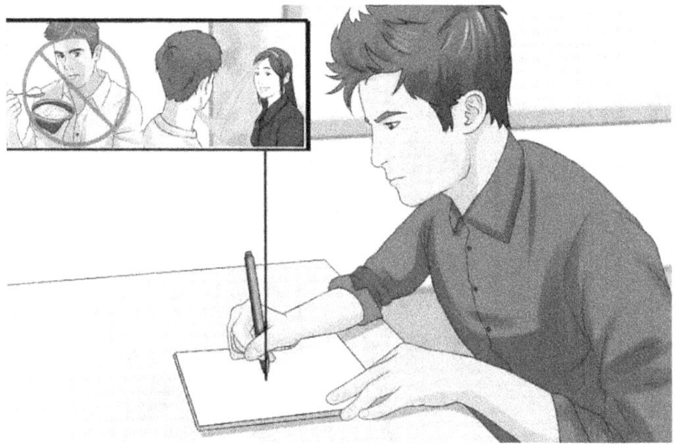

Dieting may be difficult, particularly if you are thinking hard about food and eating out of bored. Staying active and engaging in things that you like is the greatest method to suppress your hunger.

Creating a list of additional tasks to do might assist in reducing excessive snacking and boredom in eating. Keep this list ready for when the need to eat strikes.

Try going for a stroll, reading a book, clearing out a kitchen drawer, calling a friend and family member, or completing domestic tasks.

If you're hungry and it's near to a scheduled meal and snack time, eat your food and then go about your business. Continue not to eat and snack.

4. Control your tension.

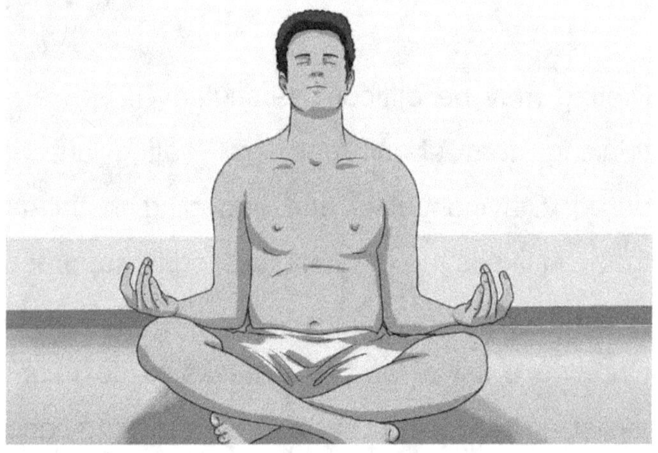

When we are under prolonged stress, our bodies produce levels of cortisol, which leads the body to retain excess fat around the waist.

Furthermore, persistently increased cortisol levels might stimulate appetite.

Try to avoid and handle stressful circumstances, people, and things in your life. Learn how to effectively handle the stress associated with unchangeable aspects of your life (like your job, for example). Talking with a personal trainer or counselor might help you find new ways to deal with stress.

Remember that although you may not always be able to control the circumstances, you can always control how you respond to them. Mind/body techniques such as yoga and meditation teach you how to calm your mind so you can manage better with tension, anxiety, and sadness.

HEALTH BENEFITS OF BELLY FAT

Both men and women are concerned about belly fat, not just for cosmetic reasons but also because of health concerns. This sort of fat covers the organs and, if it is too high, may put you at risk for cardiovascular disease, diabetes type 2, and some malignancies.

Visceral fat has also been shown to rise with age. According to research, visceral fat may grow by up to 200% in males and 400percent in women between the ages of 30 and 70. 5 Because many individuals eat 2,000 calories or more per day, a 400-600 calorie reduction on the Fat Belly Diet will almost certainly lead to weight loss.

The diet also promotes the intake of monounsaturated fats derived from plants, which have been associated with a lower risk of cardiovascular disease.

Eating more plant-based meals may also boost overall health. Plant-based diets have been linked to a lower incidence of chronic illness and obesity, according to research.

HEALTH RISK FOR BELLY FAT

Although there are no obvious health dangers linked with Belly Fat Diet, a certain study has shown that a rise in the number of meals might also mean increased daily calorie intake, which could contribute to weight gain or even a lack of weight reduction effects.

Additionally, the guarantee of a 15-pound reducing weight in 32 days is ridiculous. A healthy weight reduction pace is usually 1 to 2 pounds each week. More weight reduction would be due to water loss rather than fat loss, which isn't sustained and is not a good method to present in the form of weight control.

FOOD LIST: WHAT TO EAT AND AVOIDED

1. Mushrooms

One of the main motives mushrooms are on this list is because they are low-calorie substitutes for high-calorie items. Another explanation is that mushrooms are a naturally occurring plant-based source of vitamin D.

2. Raspberries

They're tasty and provide a splash of color to any food, whether it's a salad or a bowl of oats, but that's not all they're useful for. Raspberries are high in fiber, vitamins, and minerals including vitamin K, manganese, and C. Vitamin C boosts your immunity, while fiber keeps you fuller for longer, allowing you to eat fewer calories throughout the day. Manganese, on the other hand, has been shown to increase metabolism, which aids in the burning of belly fat.

3. Nuts

Some individuals may avoid nuts because they are heavy in calories and fat. However, if you watch your calories, you may have a few nuts in your diet without exceeding your daily calorie consumption. In terms of fat content, they are high in healthy fats that are beneficial for your heart and lower your risk of type II diabetes. Because of their high protein and fiber content, nuts are excellent weight-reduction meals that aid in the removal of belly fat. Fiber, as previously said, and protein both keep you satiated for longer. Protein goes a step further to assist raise your metabolism, allowing you to burn off more calories and 'melt' away belly fat.

4. Avocados

If you haven't already jumped on the avocado bandwagon, now is the moment. Whether you eat it on toast, in guacamole, in salads, or avocado boats, this fruit is a perfect addition to the 32 foods that burn belly fat quickly, and scientific studies back this up.

eating half an avocado at lunch lessens your urge to eat or snack later, suggesting that it may work as an appetite suppressor. This fruit's monounsaturated fats have also been proven to aid with fat and weight reduction. According to one 2013 research, those who drank 40 grams of high-oleic oils daily for four weeks lost 1.6% more belly fat than those who consumed a polyunsaturated fat-rich soil mix.

Previous research published in 2007 concluded that monounsaturated fat may prevent body fat distribution around the abdomen by down-regulating the expression of certain fat genes. All of these findings indicate that eating at least half an avocado every day may help you reduce abdominal fat.

5. Eggs

Eggs, whether boiled, poached, scrambled, or fried, are excellent weight-reduction meals. They are heavy in protein, which keeps you satiated for longer, and also contain vitamin D, which has been proven to aid with belly fat. Eggs include all nine amino acids that humans need, and studies have shown that amino acids can enhance energy metabolism, allowing you to burn calories quicker before they are converted and stored as fat.

6. Grapefruit

For good reason, this fruit has been praised as one of the finest meals for weight reduction. Studies on both animals and humans have revealed that those who eat a grapefruit every day or drink grapefruit juice lose more weight. Researchers believe that this fruit has chemicals that lower insulin levels and promote weight reduction. Instead of attempting the grapefruit juice diet, look for methods to include this fruit and its juice in a healthy, well-balanced meal.

7. Cocoa Butter

If you've done the keto diet or know anybody who has, you've probably heard about bullet coffee, which is just a cup of coffee with a tablespoon of coconut oil added to it. Coconut oil is effective for weight reduction because certain of its fatty acids may suppress hunger and stimulate fat burning. Medium-chain triglycerides (MCTs) in coconut oil are likewise swiftly and immediately absorbed into circulation. MCTs are believed to enhance a sensation of fullness, which helps you consume less food in a day. Keep in mind that coconut oil has just as many calories as any other fat and should be used in moderation.

8. Chilies

They are believed to temporarily increase your metabolism, allowing you to burn more calories and therefore lose weight and belly fat.

9. Other Nut Butters and Peanut Butter

Instead of using sweet jams and jellies to put over toast, try peanut butter (or other nut butter instead). Peanut butter may also be eaten as a snack with fruits and vegetables such as apples or celery. Natural peanut butter has up to 8 grams of protein and 4 grams of fiber per serving, which keeps you nourished for longer and increases your metabolism.

10. Oatmeal

Because of their high fiber content, oats are one of the 32 foods that burn belly fat quickly. As previously said, fiber promotes satiety, which means you eat less each day. However, oats are more than simply good for weight reduction. They are very beneficial to your general health since they reduce blood cholesterol levels, enhance the immune system, and manage blood glucose levels. To make your smoothies healthier and more satisfying, have some oats for breakfast, make some oat pancakes, or add some oat flour to them.

11. Chickpeas

Chickpeas should be on your shopping list if you want to lose belly fat, whether you are a vegan, vegetarian, or meat eater. They are a good source of plant-based protein and fiber, both of which help with fat reduction and weight loss.

12. Chocolate, dark

Dark chocolate has been touted as a superfood for good reason. It has been related in many studies to:

Enhancing insulin sensitivity (which is associated with increased weight loss and reduced fat storage)

Reduces hunger and appetite

Improves your mood, which has been shown to aid in weight reduction.

13. Salmon

It like eggs is high in omega-3 fatty acids, which aid in weight loss. It's also high in lean protein, which boosts satiety and metabolism.

14. Broccoli

Dark green vegetables, such as broccoli, were connected to lower visceral and liver fat in overweight Latino kids in a 2014 research published in the Journal of the Academy of Nutrition and Dietetics. These veggies also improved insulin sensitivity, which aids in weight reduction and lowers the risk of type II diabetes.

15. Pumpkin

Pumpkin enters our list of the 32 foods that burn belly fat quickly because of its high fiber content and low-calorie count. It not only keeps your content for longer, eliminating unhealthy eating, but it also does not interfere with your daily energy requirements.

16. Seeds of Chia

They are high in key nutrients such as omega-3s, fiber, and proteins, which assist to increase your metabolic rate and take longer to digest, keeping you content for longer and minimizing excessive snacking.

17. Cherries that are tart

Cherries are often connected with sleep since they may assist persons suffering from insomnia sleep. According to 2009 research, however, frequent eating of these fruits may aid anybody asking how to lose belly fat. The mice in the research shed weight while also lowering their hyperlipidemia, percentage fat mass, and abdominal fat.

18. Seeds of Sunflower

They are high in polyunsaturated fats, which are beneficial for your heart and lower your risk of type II diabetes. Sunflower seeds are one of the 32 foods that burn abdominal fat quickly since they are high in protein and fiber.

19. Quinoa

It is high in fiber and contains all nine necessary amino acids, making it one of the finest meals for weight reduction. According to one 2017 research, this grain reduced and decrease triglyceride levels in overweight and obese patients while also helping them lose weight and waist circumference.

20. Peas

Green peas or split peas are both excellent weight-reduction meals since they are abundant in vitamins, minerals, and fiber. They also provide complex carbs, which are an excellent source of energy. Peas are also strong in protein, which helps you feel fuller for longer and speeds up your metabolism.

21. Blueberries

A diet high in blueberries may help you lose belly fat. The mice in the research had lower levels of belly fat, triglycerides, and overall body weight. Blueberries are also abundant in vitamins that boost your immune system.

22. Beans

They, like peas, are a complex carbohydrate that provides your body with the energy it needs for extended periods. Beans are also strong in plant-based protein and carbohydrates, which increase satiety and metabolism, making them an excellent and inexpensive way to lose belly fat.

23. Milk

ilk in favor of tree alternatives, you should reconsider. Milk is one of the foods that burn belly fat quickly since it contains vitamins and minerals such as calcium and vitamin D3. According to a 2013 randomized control experiment, participants who supplemented their calorie-restricted diet using 600 mg basic iron or 125 IU vitamin D3 shed greater visceral fat and total body fat than those who did not.

24. Yogurt

Dairy products such as plain or Greek yogurt, like milk, are among the healthiest foods for weight reduction, high-protein snacks like yogurt are excellent for losing belly fat because they help manage your appetite, counteract hunger, and reduce your total food consumption.

25. Red bell peppers

Bell peppers are excellent weight loss foods because they are high in critical minerals, vitamins, and antioxidants, which aid in illness prevention and weight reduction. However, it is a chemical called capsaicin that has been discovered to improve the fat-burning rate and reduce hunger, which may assist in weight reduction, that has landed them on our list of 32 foods that burn belly fat quickly.

26. Apples

Consuming apples, whether chopped in a salad, eaten whole, or included in a morning smoothie, is one approach to eliminating belly fat. Fruit contains unsolid acid, a molecule that stimulates metabolism, boosts brown fat (the good fat) and helps prevent diet-induced obesity.

27. Tea

Because of the presence of catechins, this drink enters the list of the top 32 foods that burn belly fat quickly whether you drink green tea, black tea, or oolong tea. Catechins have long been lauded for their potential fat-burning and weight-loss properties. participants who ingested green tea catechins lost 0.6 kg, 1.7 kg, and 2.3 kg of lean mass, weight, and body fat mass, respectively. Green tea catechins (625mg/d) as a beverage may boost exercise-induced belly fat reduction and reduce triglyceride levels.

28. Blackberries

If tea does not work for you, you may supplement your catching consumption with blackberries. Every 100 g of blackberries has around 37 milligrams of catechins, which is approximately 14 times more than a 3/4 cup of green tea.

29. Turmeric

This spice may stain your hands and utensils, but it could help you lose that muffin top. Certain test-tube studies suggest that turmeric's major active component, curcumin, may help reduce some inflammatory indicators associated with obesity.

30. Farro

Farro is another wonderful wholegrain choice if you're bored of eating quinoa and brown rice all the time. It is abundant in fiber and protein, so eating it is another excellent strategy to decrease belly fat.

31. Foods Fermented

Fermented foods like kefir, sauerkraut, kombucha, fermented or raw cheeses, raw apple cider vinegar (with the mother), kimchi (fermented cabbage), natto, miso, or tempeh are excellent for weight loss and belly fat reduction. This is due to the presence of probiotics (good bacteria such as Lactobacillus and Bifidobacterium) that have been found to help in this process.

32. The Kiwi Fruit

Because it is strong in tree fiber and probiotic bacteria, which feed the healthy bacteria that help the metabolism run correctly, this fruit rounds out a list of 32 foods that burns belly fat rapidly.

What to avoid

Sugary Drink

Many sweet beverages, such as fruit juices, sports drinks, soft drinks, and sodas, contain a lot of sugar. Because of their high sugar content, they provide the body with a large number of calories when ingested. The issue is that they do not provide the body with critical nutrients for a healthy life. The individual who drinks a lot of these beverages is probably obtaining more of their daily calorie intake from the liquid. As a result, since the individual must still consume solid food, this may result in a calorie excess.

This calorie excess may ultimately result in unwanted weight gain. Between 2015 and 2020, the Dietary Guidelines for Americans recommend reducing the number of total calories given by sugary drinks. According to the analysis, the typical American eats 17 teaspoons of sugar per day, compared to the recommended 12 teaspoons. Another research published in 2015 linked substantial weight growth in both children and adolescents to sugar intake received through sugary drinks.

Baked Products

These foods are big offenders since they are often made with a lot of sugar, particularly high fructose corn syrup. According to a 2015 study, certain people who consume fructose-containing foods have a greater desire for food and are more likely to grow hungry. Participants who ate less fructose were shown to be less hungry and eager for food.

Most baked meals are high in harmful fats, such as saturated and trans fats, trans fats have a significant role in the development of obesity in mice. The FDA has also said that removing partly hydrogenated oils from meals may lower the number of incidents of heart attacks and sudden death. Confectionery and pastries are two examples of baked foods to avoid. Foods high in nutritive sweetness and fructose, on the other hand, should be avoided at all costs.

Fries in French

If they fried your food, it was almost probably high in calories, unhealthy fats, and salt. Most restaurants and eating facilities deep fry their fries to make them crispy. The difficulty here is that such food consumes a substantial amount of calories and fat. In a 2017 study of 4,440 people aged 45 to 75 who ate a potato, it was shown that some who ingested fried cabbage at least twice per week had a greater likelihood of dying than individuals who ate the meal less often. As a consequence, it is advised to limit your consumption of French fries or other fried meals. Consuming fresh vegetables and fruits might help.

Chips and Cracker

Because of their processed character, these items are featured on this list. They are often high in calories and include fat, salt, and simple carbs. During research in Brazil, it was discovered that there was a link between obesity and fast foods. To simulate the crunchiness of chips, snack on carrots and toasted nuts.

Pasta and white bread

These meals should be avoided if you want to decrease belly fat since they are often prepared from refined wheat flour. Refined wheat flour is high in simple carbs and calories but low in other important elements like fiber and protein. Instead of this sort of pasta and bread, go for whole-grain pasta and bread. This is recommended since whole-grain wheat has a lot of fiber and other minerals. This meal also healthily fills the stomach. Whole grain wheat flours like brown rice flour and whole rye flour are healthy choices to use while attempting to lose weight.

Bars of Energy and Granola

This sort of cuisine often has a large quantity of fiber and protein, but it may also have a significant amount of sugar. Although most people like eating this sort of cuisine, it is not perfect for those who wish to lose some excess belly fat. Instead of energy and granola bars, eat diced apple and peanut butter, berries, plain Greek yogurt, and hard-boiled eggs.

Dried Fruits Sweetened

When fruits are dried, they have a high concentration of fructose. As a result, it is simple to assume that dried fruit has more sugar and calories than fresh fruit. This does not exclude you from eating dried fruits when attempting to reduce weight. The essential word is always moderation. You should also avoid eating dried fruits that have been sweetened by the addition of sugar.

Alcohol

It is generally recommended that anybody wishing to lose weight around their stomach avoid alcohol. This is due to the high calorie and sugar content of most alcoholic beverages, as well as the lack of critical nutrients required for a healthy life. According to the National Institute on Alcohol Abuse and Alcoholism, consuming a particular quantity of alcohol provides the body with more calories than is necessary for a healthy lifestyle. While trying to lose weight, you may consume some kinds of alcohol in moderation, such as red wine, as well as pure alcohol such as rum, vodka, and gin.

These legal alcoholic beverages, however, must be drunk responsibly. For example, in Dietary Guidelines for Americans, males should have no more than two cups of beverages per day, while women should consume no more than one cup per day.

Meat Processing

This sort of food is improper for you since it has gone through numerous forms of food processing in food production plants. These meats might have been fermented, canned, smoked, or dried, and they are normally packaged and preserved to have a longer shelf life. As a consequence of the preparation, these meats often have significant salt content. They lack the bulk of the important elements that the body needs to keep healthy, and they also have a high-calorie content when compared to other protein sources such as fish, beans, chicken, and so on.

Meats that have been processed in any way, according to the International Agency for Research on Cancer (IARC), are carcinogenic, which means they may cause some forms of cancer. This is to say that processed meats such as hot dogs, ham, salami, jerky, and bacon, to name a few, should be avoided if you truly want to lose belly fat.

The Ice Cream

Most ice creams are high in calories and sugar content, and sadly, this creamy delicacy has little to no protein and fiber value. The appropriate quantity of ice cream is normally half a cup; however, this advice may be ignored since it is quite simple to forget the required ratio when eating it. Instead of ice cream, try frozen fruits or some delectable combinations of Greek yogurt and chopped fruits.

RECIPE FOR BELLY FAT

Peanuts with Chile Lime

Ingredients

- 6 teaspoon lime juice
- 6 tbsp. chili powder
- 1/2-1 tsp cayenne pepper
- 1/2-1 tsp cayenne pepper

* 6 cups cocktail peanuts, unsalted

Directions

Step 1

Preheat the oven to 250°F with racks in the top and bottom thirds.

Step 2

In a large mixing bowl, combine the lime juice, chili flakes, salt, and cayenne pepper. Toss in the peanuts to coat. Divide the mixture evenly between two large-rimmed baking sheets.

Step 3

Bake for 45 minutes, stirring after 15 minutes, until dry. Allow cooling fully. Keep it in a sealed container.

Lemony-Parsley Pesto Chickpea Pasta

Ingredients

- 4 oz. chickpea penne or even other macaroni noodles (about 1 1/4 cups dry)
- 1 bunch plain cilantro (about 4 cups gently packed), plus additional for garnish
- 3 garlic cloves
- 1/3 cup virgin olive oil
- 2 tablespoons lime juice 1 teaspoon lemon juice
- 1/2 tsp kosher salt 14 tsp crushed black pepper
- 1 pound roasted root veggies (see associated recipe)

Directions

Step 1

Cook the pasta according to the package instructions. Drain thoroughly.

Step 2

Meanwhile, in a food processor, mix parsley and garlic and pulse until evenly chopped, approximately 10 times. Add the oil, lemon juice, salt, and pepper and blend for approximately 15 seconds, or until just incorporated; it should be chunky.

Step 3

Microwave roasted veggies in a microwave-safe dish for 1 minute, or until heated through. (Alternatively, in a large pan over medium-high heat, heat 1 tsp extra-virgin olive oil.) Cook, turning often, until veggies are cooked throughout, 2 to 4 mins.)

Step 4

Combine the heated pasta, pesto, veggies, and lemon zest in a large mixing bowl. If desired, garnish with parsley.

Salad of Chickpeas, Artichokes, and Avocado with Apple-Cider Dressing

Ingredients

- 2 tbsp. apple cider vinegar
- 2 tsp whole-grain mustard
- 1 tablespoon shallot chopped
- 1/4 teaspoon salt 14 teaspoons pepper
- 1/4 cup additional olive oil
- 8 cups salad greens, mixed (about 5 ounces)
- 1 (1/4 oz.) can of washed and halved and quartered artichoke hearts
- 1 cup drained, salt-free chickpeas
- 1 avocado, diced
- 2 eggs, hard-boiled

Directions

Step 1

In a large mixing bowl, combine vinegar, vinegar, shallot, salt, and pepper. Whisk in the oil until smooth. Salad greens, artichokes, chickpeas, and avocados are optional. Grate the eggs into the bowl using a box grater with big holes. Gently toss to mix.

Omelets in Muffin Tins with Feta and Peppers

Ingredients

- Spray cooking oil
- 2 tbsp. extra virgin olive oil
- 3/4 cup chopped onion
- 1/4 teaspoon salt, divided 1 medium diced red bell pepper
- 1 tablespoon fresh oregano, finely chopped
- 8 medium eggs
- 3/4 cup feta cheese, crumbled
- 1/2 cup skim milk
- 1/2 teaspoon black pepper

- 1/4 cup chopped Kalamata olives 2 cups minced fresh spinach

Directions

Step 1

Preheat the oven to 325°F. Coat a 12-cup cupcake pan well with cooking spray.

Step 2

In some kind of a large skillet on medium-high heat, heat the oil. Cook, stirring constantly until the onion begins to soften, approximately 3 minutes. Cook, stirring occasionally until the veggies are soft and beginning skillet brown, 4 to 5 minutes longer. Remove from the fire and set aside for 5 minutes to cool.

Step 3

In a large mixing bowl, combine the eggs, feta, milk, and pepper, as well as the additional 1/8 teaspoon salt. Mix in the spinach, olives, and vegetable combination. Divide the mixture among the prepped muffin cups.

Step 4

Bake for 25 minutes, or until hard to the touch. Allow for a 5-minute rest before taking from the tin.

Salad of Spinach and Artichoke with Parmesan Vinaigrette

Ingredients

- 1 can (15 oz.) quartered artichoke hearts
- a single recipe Vinaigrette with Parmesan (see Associated Recipes)
- 1 package (5 ounces) of baby greens (about 6 cups)
- 6 eggs, hard-boiled
- 1/4 cup unsalted chopped pistachios

Directions

Step 1

Using towels and perhaps a clean dish towel, line a sheet pan. Drain artichokes in a wire-mesh strainer then rinse well with cold water before draining again. Set aside. Arrange chopped artichokes in a thin layer just on the prepared pan (to eliminate moisture).

Step 2

Divide the vinaigrette evenly into four small covered containers.

Step 3

Divide the artichokes into four individual serving containers. Top each with a quarter of the spinach. Freeze for up to four days after sealing the containers.

Step 4

Slice 1 1/2 difficult eggs and put them in the food container in the mornings before packing your lunch. Just before serving, drizzle with the vinaigrette and top with 1 tablespoon of pistachios.

Chole (Chickpea Curry) (Chickpea Curry)

Ingredients

- 1 medium promotes higher pepper, quartered
- 4 big garlic cloves
- 1 peeled and finely chopped 2-inch piece of grated ginger
- 1 medium sliced yellow onion (1-inch)
- 6 tablespoons grapeseed or canola oil
- 2 tablespoons coriander powder
- 2 tablespoons cumin powder
- 1/2 teaspoon turmeric powder
- 1/4 cup canned pureed tomatoes with liquid, no salt added (from a 28-ounce can)

- a quarter teaspoon of kosher salt
- 2 rinsed 15-ounce cans of chickpeas
- 2 tablespoons garam masala
- Garnish with fresh cilantro

Directions

Step 1

In a food processor, mince the serrano, garlic, and ginger. Scrape the sides down and pulse once more. Add the onion and pulse until it is coarsely minced but not watery.

Step 2

In a large saucepan, heat the oil over medium-high heat. Cook, stirring periodically until the onion mixture is cooked, 3 to 5 minutes. Stir in the coriander, cumin, and turmeric for 2 minutes.

Step 3

In a food processor, pulse tomatoes until finely chopped. Add to the pan with the salt. Reduce the heat to retain a simmering and cook for 4 minutes, stirring periodically. Reduce heat to a medium simmer, add chickpeas, and cook for 5 minutes longer, stirring periodically. If desired, garnish with cilantro.

"Donuts" made from apples

Ingredients

- 1 large apple
- 3 tbsp. almond butter
- 2 teaspoons unsweetened shredded coconut

Directions

Step 1

Using an apple coring tool, remove the apple core. Cut the apple into 8 thin rings, approximately 1/4 inch thick, crosswise. Spread almond butter on each apple ring. Coat with coconut.

Latte with Matcha Green Tea

Ingredients

- 1/4 cup hot water
- 1 teaspoon powdered matcha tea
- 1 cup skim milk
- 1 tablespoon honey

Directions

Step 1

In a blender, combine hot water and matcha powder until frothy. Heat the milk and honey until nearly boiling. Whisk the milk vigorously until it is foamy. Put the milk into a cup, followed by the tea.

Avocado Toast with Everything Bagel

Ingredients

- 1/4 medium mashed avocado

* 1 toasted piece of whole-grain bread
* 2 tablespoons of everything bagel seasoning
* 1 tsp flaky kosher salt (such as Malden)

Directions

Step 1: Spread the avocado on the bread. Season with salt and pepper to taste.

Avocado Pesto Noodles Squash & Chicken

Ingredients

* 1 spaghetti squash, split lengthwise and seeded,
* 2 1/2 to 3 pounds
* 1 avocado, ripe
* 1 cup basil leaves, packed
* 1/4 cup shelled pistachios, unsalted
* 2 tbsp. of lemon juice
* 1 garlic clove

- 1 pound armless, skinless chicken breast, cut and chopped into 1-inch pieces,
- 3/4 teaspoon salt,
- 1/2 teaspoon powdered pepper,
- 5 tablespoons extra-virgin olive oil

Directions

Step 1

Preheat the oven to 400°F. Cooking spray a big-rimmed baking sheet.

Step 2

Arrange the squash solely on a single side of a prepared pan, and cut the side down. Bake for 45 minutes, or until the potatoes are soft.

Step 3

Meanwhile, in a food processor, blend avocado, basil, walnuts, lime juice, onion, 1/2 teaspoon salt, and 1/4 teaspoon pepper. Pulse until everything is finely chopped. 4 tablespoons oil, process until smooth

Step 4

Toss the chicken with the remaining 1 tablespoon oil and 1/4 teaspoon salt and pepper in a medium bowl for ten minutes first before the squash is done. Place the chicken in a uniform layer on the baking sheet's empty side. Return to the oven and bake for 10 minutes, or until just cooked through.

Step 5

Scrape the squash from the shells into a large mixing dish using a fork. Toss in the chicken carefully to integrate. Serve with pesto on top.

Salad with White Beans and Veggies

Ingredients

* 2 cups salad greens, mixed

- 3/4 cup chopped vegetables of your choice, such as cucumbers and cherry tomatoes
- 13 cups rinsed and drained canned white beans
- 12 diced avocado
- 1 tbsp. red wine vinegar
- 2 tsp extra virgin olive oil
- 14 tsp kosher salt
- To taste, freshly ground pepper

Directions

Step 1 In a medium mixing bowl, combine the greens, vegetables, beans, and avocado. Season with salt and pepper and drizzle with vinegar and oil. Toss everything together and transfer it to a big platter.

Paulist a Shrimp

Ingredients

- 2 pounds big peeled and deveined shrimp
- 2 teaspoon lime juice
- 1/2 cup chopped fresh cilantro, 8 minced garlic cloves,
- 1/2 teaspoon kosher salt,
- 1/2 teaspoon crushed red pepper,
- 2 tablespoons extra-virgin olive oil

Directions

Step 1

Toss shrimp with lime juice, 1/4 cup parsley, half the onion, 1/4 teaspoon salt, and 1/4 teaspoon chopped red pepper in a medium nonstick bowl. Refrigerate the marinade for 20 minutes, covered.

Step 2

In a large skillet on medium-high heat, heat the oil. Cook till the shrimp just are cooked through, approximately 5 minutes, with the shrimp, marinade, and remaining garlic. Remove from the fire and stir in the remaining 1/4 cup cilantro, 1/4 teaspoon salt, and 1/4 teaspoon red pepper flakes. To mix, toss everything together.

Toast with white beans and avocado

Ingredients

- 1 slice whole-wheat loaf, toasted
- 1/4 avocado, mashed
- 1/2 cup canned white beans, washed and drained
- to taste, ground pepper
- 1 pinch of Red pepper, crushed

Directions

Step 1 Spread diced avocado with white beans on bread. Season with salt, pepper, and chopped red pepper to taste.

MEAL PLAN

Day 1

Breakfast: Make an omelet without egg yolks. Mix in a handful of greens and 75g of chopped mixed peppers.

Mid-morning snack: 100 grams of grilled chicken with 1/2 slice of red pepper

Lunch: 1/4 tbsp. olive oil grilled chicken breast On the side, serve with black beans, red peppers, or assorted salad leaves.

Afternoon snack: 100g grilled chicken breast with 14 slices of cucumber

Dinner: Broccoli steamed on roasted chicken (100 grams).

Day 2

Breakfast: Cook a handful of greens in a skillet and serve with roasted chicken breast.

Mid-morning snack: 12 sliced green pepper, 100 g of fresh turkey breast

Lunch: 1/2 tablespoon olive oil served with a mix of green salad and roasted haddock fillet

Afternoon snack: 100g grilled turkey breast with 75g steamed broccoli

Dinner: Steamed green beans with a salmon fillet and chopped dill

Day 3

Breakfast: smoked salmon with a handful of green spinach (100 grams).

Mid-morning snack: 1/2 yellow pepper slices and 100 g chicken breast

Lunch: 1/2 yellow peppers marinated in 1/2 tablespoon olive oil on 100 g of chicken breast.

Afternoon snack: 1/4 avocado slices placed atop 100 grams of roasted turkey slices

Dinner: With two cutlets, steamed spinach, and broccoli (or one lamb steak, grilled).

Day 4

Breakfast: Tomatoes, two poached eggs (two whites and one whole), and green beans.

Mid-morning snack: 14 sliced cucumbers with 100 g turkey slices

Lunch: Baked cod fillet with greens, tomato, salad, and 1/2 tbsp. olive oil

Afternoon snack: 12 grilled courgettes, 100 g chicken breast

Dinner: Medium-heat chicken breast (100 g) with green vegetables and 1/2 tbsp. olive oil

Day 5

Breakfast: 200g grilled turkey breast with 14 slices cucumber and 14 avocado

Mid-morning snack:

1/2 slices red pepper marinated atop two hard-boiled eggs

Lunch: Grilled prawns (150g), tomato, green salad, and 1/2 tbsp. olive oil

Afternoon snack: Turkey breast with five almonds (100 grams)

Dinner: Broccoli steamed with chicken chest (100 grams)

Day 6

Breakfast: Roasted peppers with a grilled haddock fillet and a sprinkle of zucchini

Mid-morning snack: 100 grams of cooked chicken and one sliced tomato

Lunch: Steamed broccoli with 1/2 tbsp. olive oil and 150g turkey, accented with a green salad

Afternoon snack: 5 pecan nuts per 100g of chicken

Dinner: Steak (150-200g) with broccoli with green beans (steamed).

Day 7

Breakfast: Three omelets with cooked spinach with roasted tomatoes (egg whites only).

Mid-morning snack: For 100 grams of turkey, combine five Brazil nuts.

Lunch: Asparagus steamed with a simple salad and 150g chicken breast

Afternoon snack: 1/4 sliced cucumber with 100 g turkey

Dinner: Skinless duck breast with cauliflower (or cooked oriental greens) (grilled).

CONCLUSION

Belly fat is among the most difficult fats to lose. To get treatment for stubborn belly fat, you need a long-term, healthy regimen. Making simple adjustments in your life may have a big impact on your total weight and belly fat. A rise in belly fat may suggest a variety of health concerns, including diabetes, heart disease, and liver damage. Men's and women's bodies react differently to abdominal fat. While belly fat in males causes cardiovascular disease, disease resistance, and high blood pressure, Harvard Health Publishing reports that belly fat in women is more dangerous. A hip-to-waist and BMI study reveals that women had an 18% higher likelihood of having a heart attack than males. In women, it may also raise the risk of developing diabetes and breast cancer.

www.ingramcontent.com/pod-product-compliance
Lightning Source LLC
Chambersburg PA
CBHW071224260726

48653CB00042B/2001